Teen Sexuality Resources

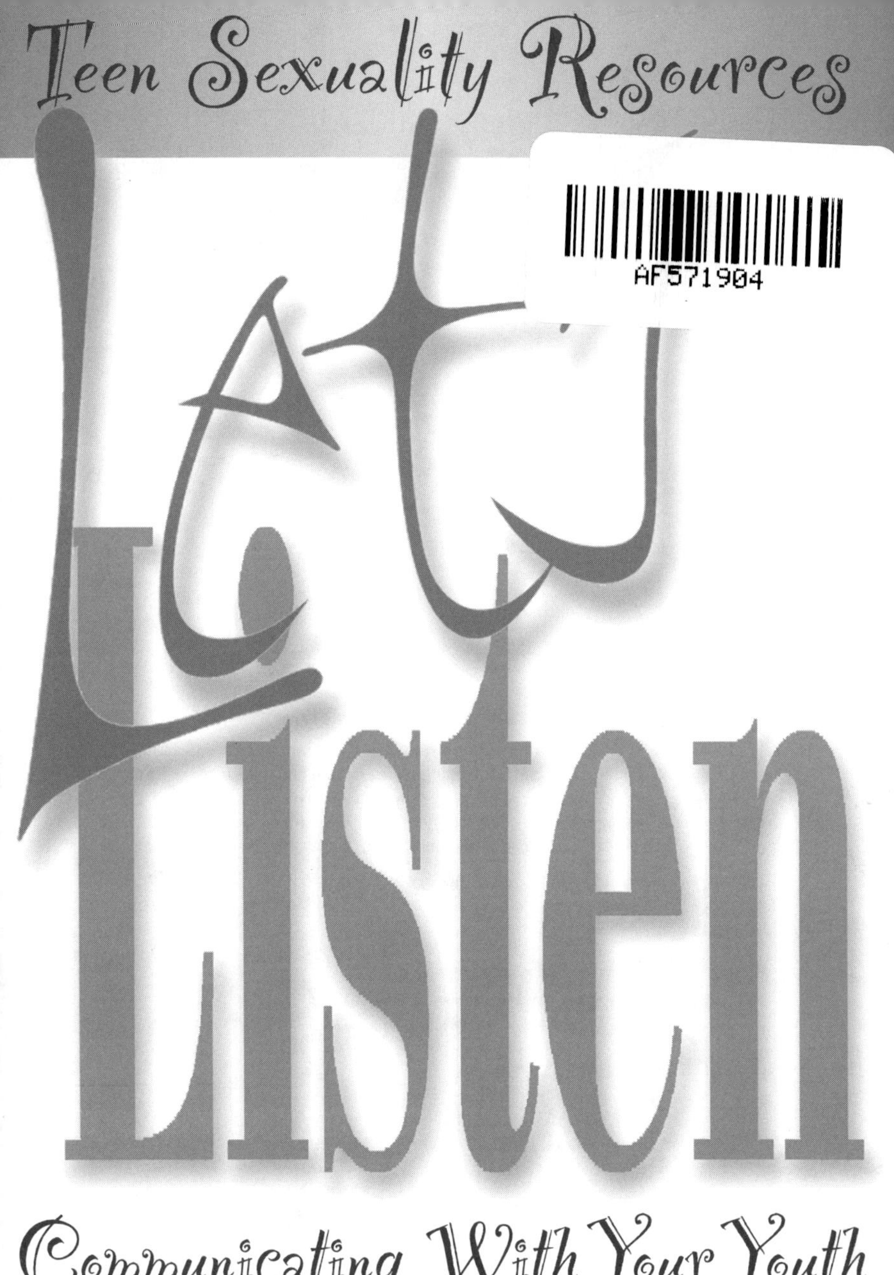

Communicating With Your Youth About Faith and Sexuality

Parent Resource

Let's Listen: Communicating With Your Youth About Faith and Sexuality

(ISBN 0-687-72215-2)

EDITORIAL AND DESIGN TEAM
Duane A Ewers and M. Steven Games, *Editors*
Phillip D. Francis, *Designer*

ADMINISTRATIVE TEAM
Neil M. Alexander, *Publisher*
Harriett Jane Olson, *Vice President*
Duane A. Ewers, *Executive Editor, Teaching and Study Resources*
M. Steven Games, *Senior Editor of Youth Resources*

Cover design by Phillip D. Francis

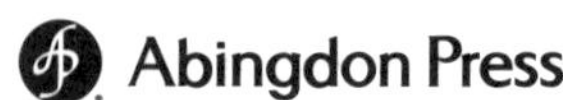

THIS PUBLICATION IS PRINTED ON RECYCLED PAPER.

03 04 05 06 07—10 9

PURPOSE

To help parents and youth have honest discussions about beliefs, values, and sexuality so that youth have guidance in their faith journey and their decision-making.

Table of Contents

Introduction 4
The Most Important Person in the Room

Session 1 6
Media and Images of Faith

Session 2 9
Listen to Your Body

Session 3 14
What to Do? Positive Christian Decision-making

Session 4 20
They're in Too Deep! Positive Christian Relationships

Session 5 24
Wait, Wait, Wait It Out!

Session 6 27
Big-Button Issues: How Could I Possibly Talk to My Teen About That!

Conclusion 32
Final Exam

Introduction: The Most Important Person in the Room

Let's listen in on a conversation between Justin, a teenager, and his dad (who could be you).

Justin: "Jessica has slept with every guy on the football team! She's a slut. I'll never date a slut!"

Justin has just said something important about himself. What will Dad say that will keep the focus of the conversation on Justin? Is Jessica or Justin the most important person at this moment in time? Does the parent defend Jessica's honor, trying to sort out truth from rumor and exaggeration? Or does he pursue the values that Justin has expressed?

Dad: "How do you know it's true?"

Where does the conversation go next? Jessica's virtue has become the topic, not Justin's beliefs and value system. He has shared some important information about himself. He has told you that values, image, and reputation are important to him. Now, do you want to defend Jessica, or find out what Justin believes?

If you are reading this book, you probably have a youth in a human sexuality learning experience in your congregation. Your teens will be encouraged to talk with you about faith, values, sexuality, and decision-making. **LET'S LISTEN is about helping parents listen to teens so teens will talk and so they will also listen.** Listening to one another is crucial when trying to communicate about important issues. You, the parent, are more likely to be heard if you listen first. When you talk to your youth, remember that he or she is the most important person in the room.

This resource will be Christian and biblical in its focus. Turn to Luke 10:25-28, and listen to God's Word: "An expert in the Law of

Moses stood up and asked Jesus a question to see what he would say. 'Teacher,' he asked, 'what must I do to have eternal life?' "

Of course Jesus knows the answer, but the most important person in the room is the "expert" who needs to learn something about himself and his motivations. Jesus bounces the question back to him. "Jesus answered, 'What is written in the Scriptures? How do you understand them?' The man replied, 'The Scriptures say, "Love the Lord your God with all your heart, soul, strength, and mind." They also say, "Love your neighbors as much as you love yourself." ' " Jesus said, 'You have given the right answer.' "

Return to the imaginary conversation with your teen. Maybe he is testing your ability to listen. Using Jesus' approach, what would you say to the teen?

Possible answer: "Why wouldn't you date a slut?" The focus of the question shifts back to Justin. The youth must wrestle with the answer, not you. Do you know the answer? Probably. But you want your son to think for himself, so give him the chance to answer. You'll discover something about his values and his maturity. Listen to your teen!

Too often we believe that conversations with our youth are about telling them what to think and what to do, when the real task involves listening to them and hearing what they are saying. By listening we help teens explore their own understandings of their beliefs and values that relate to sexuality. Stating our values does help because they need that input from adults. However, just as you probably prefer to make a final decision on your own, rather than just accepting what someone tells you, so do your teens.

Our Theological Common Ground

We are Christian parents, so our perspective on human sexuality reflects our beliefs and values. Our values are grounded in the Christian faith, the community of faith, and the teachings of the church. Our faith finds its primary source in the Bible. The Bible is basic to talking about sexuality. Sexuality is important to the Bible, too. Genesis, the first book, in the first chapter, affirms God's good gift of sexuality. Human sexuality is a part of the creation that God declared "very good." We will want to keep our faith perspective in our conversations with youth.

1 Media and Images of Faith

Every generation has its concerns. One of the largest concerns for those entering the Third Millennium is the impact of media.

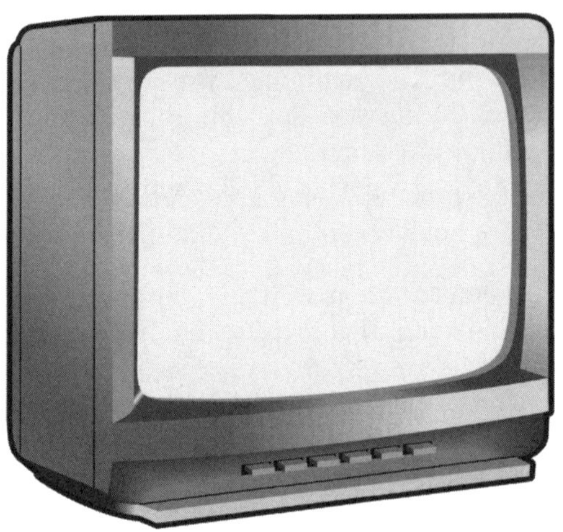

Parents all over the country have legitimate concerns about what comes across the television screen, what's shown at the movies, what's heard on the radio and on CDs, and now what is seen and read over the Internet. We have more guidelines than ever before, but little actual control. We may be able to block access to pornography in our own homes but not in the homes of our friends and neighbors. Perhaps they have different standards and values. Even so, it is important to know that we can take steps to limit our teens' exposure to pornography. We can control what happens in our living rooms.

God's Say: Images of Faith

The Christian faith is counter to the media and to the secular culture.

• The Ten Commandments remind us, "Do not tell lies about others. Do not want anything that belongs to someone else. Don't

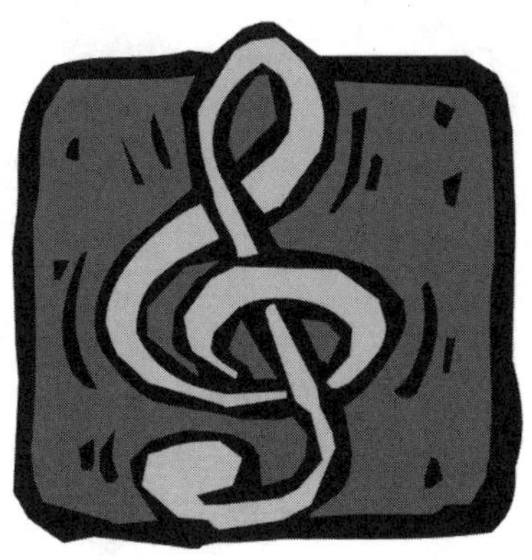

want anyone's house, wife or husband,. . . or anything else" (Exodus 20:16-17).

•However, the media bear false witness about sex appeal and attraction: "Wear this fragrance; wear these clothes; look this way; act this way to be cool and to attract the opposite sex."

•Media bear false witness about life in the real world. The media appeal to and exploit our covetous nature. We end up wanting what everyone else seems to have.

•The Bible teaches that we are created by God and are "very good" (Genesis 1:26, 31). That is, we are valued and are not to be exploited.

The church teaches that sexual relations are clearly affirmed only in the marriage bond. Abstinence is seen as a normal, valid, appropriate, healthy, and faithful choice in the midst of a culture that perpetuates the lie that everyone is "doing it." Abstinence in sexual relations is not simply a holdover from the Victorian age. It is a way of valuing other persons and oneself. It is a way to avoid "using" other persons for one's own pleasure. It is a way to prepare for the special covenant relationship with another in marriage that is God's ideal. In addition, abstinence is a way to avoid unwanted pregnancies and sexually-transmitted infections.

(Note: *Let's Decide*, the youth resource, contains Bible references and comments about abstinence similar to the ones in this resource for parents.)

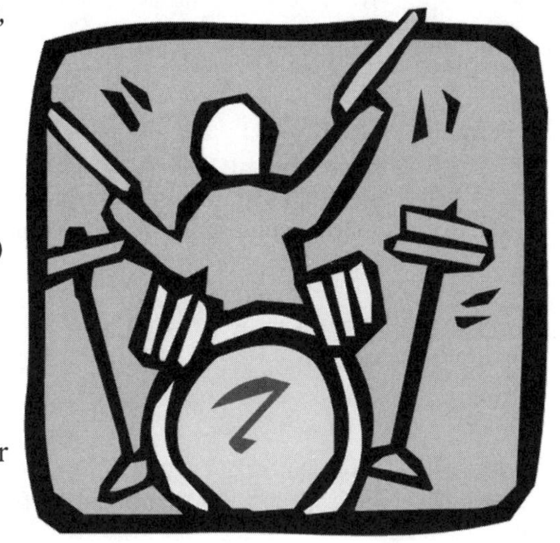

Capture the Moment

Listen! Listen to the radio, the TV, the CD player. If you hear something you don't like, let your teens know. Also point out things that are positive. Use these moments as opportunities for dialogue. Repeat what you heard. Ask: "What do you think about that?" or "What do you like about that?" Allow teens to express their views while you listen, really listen. Briefly give your views after they have commented. (Just be sure to avoid turning your comments into a lecture.)

You have let them know where you stand.

Your teens are going to get an education one way or another. They are curious; they want answers. Do you want the media to do the job for you? Does MTV know best? Be a model for the faith and provide an alternative to the media's message. Be ready to share the beliefs, images, and values that are important to you Remember, you are the parent. At times it might be necessary to refuse to allow certain programs or movies to be shown in your home. Take a stand against the media and be clear about your values. Your youth may still see these same shows when they visit their friends, but you have let them know where you stand.

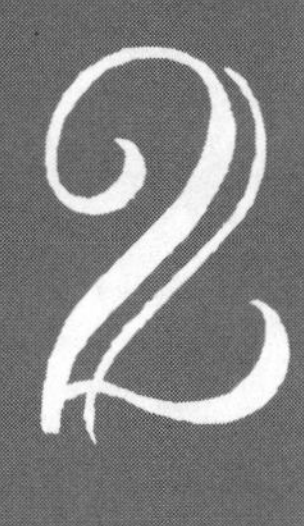

Listen to Your Body

Reflections

How do you, as a parent, feel about your body? your genitals? How did you feel about them as a teenager? Do you remember the time Mr. Lattimore called you up to the front of the class and you had an erection you were trying to hide? What are you teaching your teen about the body, not so much by what you say, but by how you act toward your body, your spouse's body, and toward bodies on TV, at the beach, or at the mall? Take a moment to write your reflections about these questions.

God's Say

"Late one afternoon, David got up from a nap and was walking around.... A beautiful young woman was down below in her courtyard, bathing as her religion required. David happened to see her, and he sent one of his servants to find out who she was.... David sent some messengers to bring her to his palace. She came to him, and he slept with her" (2 Samuel 11:2-4).

"One day [Noah] got drunk and was lying naked in his tent. Ham entered the tent and saw him naked, then went back outside and told his brothers. Shem and Japheth put a robe over their shoulders and walked backward into the tent. Without looking at their father, they placed it over his body. When Noah woke up and learned what his youngest son Ham had done, he said, 'I now put a curse on [him]!'" (Genesis 9:20-25).

Other Scriptures present a healthier view of the body than the lust and shame respectively experienced by David and Ham:

"You are the one who put me together
inside my mother's body,
and I praise you
because of the wonderful way you created me....
But with your own eyes
you saw my body being formed" (Psalm 139:13-14a, 16).

Like David and Noah, we too sometimes struggle with lust and shame. If we keep in mind that our body is God's creation, we can overcome some of those feelings. As parents we ought to affirm a healthy view of the body, rather than harboring negative feelings such as shame or lust. Viewing other people as sex objects or things is, of course, harmful and not in keeping with God's purpose for our sexuality. A sense of shame might be useful only with regard to keeping us from behaving inappropriately. However, when we talk with our teens, it is important to emphasize a positive, Christian understanding of the body.

Capture the Moment

Be familiar with the correct terms for various body parts. Say the difficult words out loud—*penis, vagina, sexual intercourse*—until they are as easy for you to say as *finger* and *arm*. Your teen will appreciate the honesty. Secure a copy of the developmental sequence in *Let's Be Real*, pages 45–52, from the leader. Stay ahead of the development of your teen. Prior to the beginning of puberty in your child, get an education about this stage of development (see pages 10–13 in *Let's Decide*) so that you can provide information to your teen about what is happening to his or her body.

More than likely you taught your children numbers and the alphabet before they started school. You may have taught them how to throw and catch before you registered them for little league. You probably taught them the primary colors before they could produce art. Understanding anatomy is the first step toward understanding sexuality. Give your teens the words and the facts that will help them understand their body. Teach your child about nocturnal emissions and menstruation before they happen.

When attempting to communicate with youth, you have several choices. You can allow any anxiety you have about your body to color all you say about sexuality. Or you can set aside your own anxiety and help your teens deal with their anxiety about their body. Just remember that the most important person is your teen.

Are you unsure of your facts because of poor communication with your own parent? Explore resources that will help you learn more about this topic. Read a book. Encourage your church leaders to have a sexuality seminar and then be sure to attend. (*Let's Be Real* is the leader resource for sexuality seminars.) Pass along pertinent information to your teen. Will your youth ever admit to needing sexuality education? Probably not. Who has the maturity or judgment to make such a decision? You do. You are the parent.

How do you begin a conversation on the topic of sexuality? It might happen in the car. It might happen as you watch TV. Your youth might initiate it. It might happen on a quiet Sunday afternoon. It might happen on the way home from the church after a human sexuality seminar. It might happen because a question is asked about Aunt Cheryl's pregnancy. It might happen when your teen questions you about a certain slang or curse word, or uses the slang or curse word. Can you think of some times when you could have captured the moment for communication?

Possible responses to opportunities to talk with your teen:

"Well, let's talk about it" or "I've been wondering how to bring that up."

"Of course, that word shocks me; but I'm more curious about what you think it means."

"We've all been worried about Aunt Cheryl's pregnancy. Do you have questions about it?"

What other responses might you use when your teen presents you with an opportunity for communication?

If your teen doesn't bring up the topic of sexuality, you might create a relaxed time to ask what she or he thinks about a certain related issue. Even if your youth is a bit uncomfortable with discussing such matters, it is important for him or her to know that you are willing to talk about the topic.

Set a positive tone. Conversations about sexuality are important. Acknowledge your feelings of nervousness, but realize that nervousness is not all you are feeling. You are also glad to have the opportunity to talk about something important to you and your teen. Let Psalm 139:13-14 be your guide instead of shame or fear:

> "You are the one who put me together
>   inside my mother's body,
> and I praise you
>   because of the wonderful way you created me."

Getting Specific

In one of her columns, Erma Bombeck repeated a conversation with her fifteen-year-old son. Erma: "I need to talk to you about sex." His response was, "Sure, Mom. What do you need to know?" Our youth can seem self-assured; but they are as uncertain as you were at their age, and are now. Do not let the media or bragging on your youth's part fool you. Teens do not know it all.

Generally, anatomy questions need straight-forward, factual answers. Opinion questions, decision-making questions, or value statements by your youth need different responses. We will look at those in the next session.

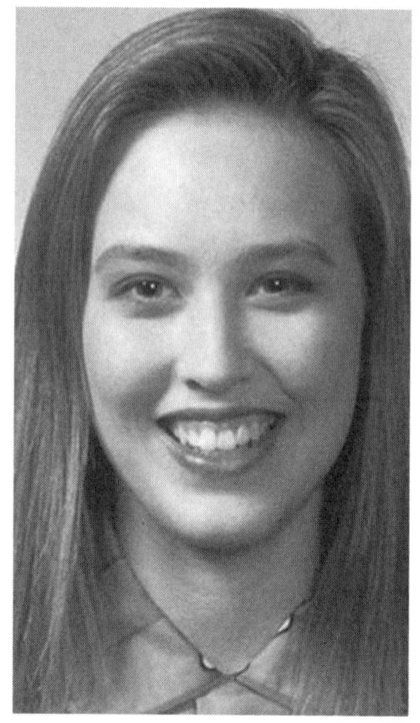

Talk about both male and female anatomy. Teens need information about the opposite sex and their own body for further discussions about values and decision-making. Your comfort level in talking about the opposite sex models an appropriate comfort level for your youth. The comparison might help their understanding of male and female emotional differences, too. You will also help relieve their anxiety by letting them know that other teens are going through similar changes.

The conversation might begin with a discussion of puberty: "What changes have you noticed in your body? Puberty is the

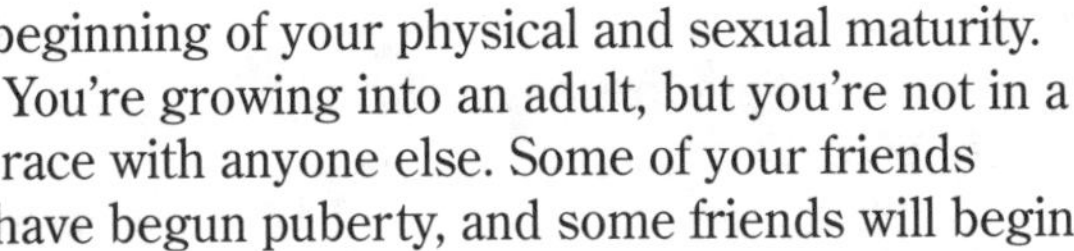

beginning of your physical and sexual maturity. You're growing into an adult, but you're not in a race with anyone else. Some of your friends have begun puberty, and some friends will begin later. We each have our own built-in alarm clock that goes off when our body is ready. Puberty usually happens between ages thirteen and fifteen; but sometimes it starts as early as nine or ten, or as late as sixteen or seventeen. Your body has its own schedule, and you can't slow it down or speed it up."

Tips for Listening

A conversation about anatomy can be a foundation for further teaching and learning.

Be comfortable with your own body.

Get an education through this book or another one, a video, or a seminar.

If you have already been talking with your teen about the body, then future conversations simply elaborate on the same subject.

Remember that the most important person in the room is your teen, not you. Squelch your own anxiety.

Don't be in a hurry to give all the information in one conversation. Just as changes in the human body are gradual, take your time when communicating with your teens.

If your son or daughter wants to know whether something happened to you, try to give an honest response. Such honesty is the best way to become a trusted adult.

Psalm 139 assures us, "You are the one who put me together inside my mother's body." The Bible lets us know that we are God's creation ("You . . . put me together"). The Bible is honest about our origin. Surely you can be honest, too, with your teen.

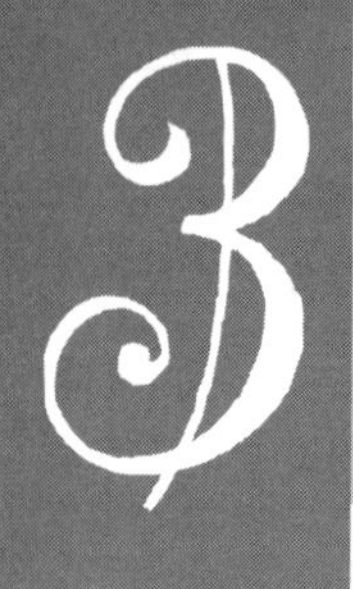

What to Do? Positive Christian Decision-making

God's Say

Read 2 Samuel 11:2-4.

Just as David gave in to his impulses with Bathsheba, some teens end up having sexual intercourse without thinking or deciding about it ahead of time. They simply succumb to opportunities that present themselves.

Note that God does not appear in the above Scripture. God's part in this decision is absent. David's decision-making is not grounded in God's values or word. Christian decision-making begins with God. God does not sanction premarital sexual intercourse (or adultery), not because God wants to be mean and restrictive, but because "No!" is sometimes best for us. God wants us to protect ourselves from disease and death and inappropriate pregnancies. God also wants us to protect ourselves spiritually and emotionally. When we engage in sexual intercourse outside marriage, we run a much greater risk of hurting ourselves and others. God protects us with the gifts of virginity and abstinence. God wants us to keep our body and soul intact and healthy.

Jesus reflects this understanding of spiritual protection when he says, "You know the commandment which says, 'Be faithful in marriage.' But I tell you that if you look at another woman and want her, you are already unfaithful in your thoughts" (Matthew 5:27-28). Jesus knew that one's thoughts, emotions, and spiritual state all relate to the realm of sexual activity.

Let's be candid about the spiritual aspects of sex as well as the physical processes that are involved. You can damage your body or conceive a child with premarital sexual intercourse, but you may also damage your soul. Which damage is greater? The answer is, of course, that both kinds of trauma are serious. Because as Jesus knew, we are a unity of body and soul. God's Word helps us make decisions that reflect this unity with regard to our sexuality.

Slowing Down the Ever-Ready Teen

Little thought goes into many teens' decisions about sexual activity. Christian decision-making means that other voices such as God's, the church's, and the parent's, will enter the dialogue in the teen's mind. Before the teen is home alone, before he or she is in the back seat of a vehicle, or before the teen is unsupervised at a party, he or she thinks through the consequences of premarital sexual intercourse or intimate sexual play.

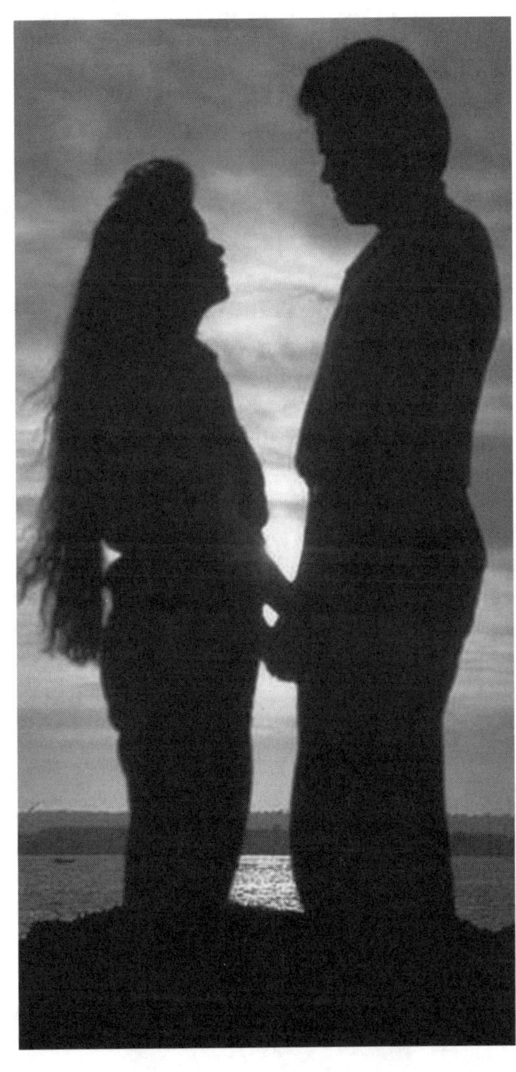

Ways to Bring Up the Subject

Be prepared to capture the moment. Unlike conversations about facts and information, conversations about values and decision-making are best initiated by the teen. But teens have a code for bringing up the subject. Pay attention to codes.

The next section gives you a chance to think about your responses to some examples of teens' broaching the subject of sexual values and decision-making.

Teen Codes and Your Response

"Jessica is a slut."
"Jason and Megan are having sex."
"What do I say to my friend who wants to have sex with his girlfriend?"
"Sarah is pregnant. What do I say to her?"

Usually the response that first leaps to a parent's mind involves trying to determine the facts in a specific case.

Parent to teen: "How do you know that?"

Does such a response focus on your teen, or the other person? Another possible response involves defending the honor of the other person. Would you be likely to answer in this manner?

Parent to teen: "You shouldn't talk about your friend like that" or "Do you know what the word *slut* means?"

Remember that your teen is the most important person in the room. Try to lay aside any possible anxiety on your part. Do you worry about Megan's and Jason's virtue? Yes, but you lay aside that concern for the moment, because **your teen and his or her viewpoints are what matter most during this conversation.**

Remember that your teen is the most important person in the room.

Teens often have indirect ways of revealing their values. Listen carefully in order to understand what they are telling you about themselves. You may discover that their values are quite similar to your own.

At other times teens are more direct about discussing their values and decisions related to sex. They may initiate a conversation having to do with sexual behavior.

More often than not, your teen will talk in code. It might happen while he or she is watching TV, with you in the car, or when she or he is doing household chores. In other words, whenever and wherever you are with teens, listen for the code.

Positive Ways to Respond to the Code

Andy: "Jessica is a slut."

How would you respond? (Remember that Andy's attitudes and beliefs are what you want to discover just now.)

Parent: "Why do you say that about Jessica?"

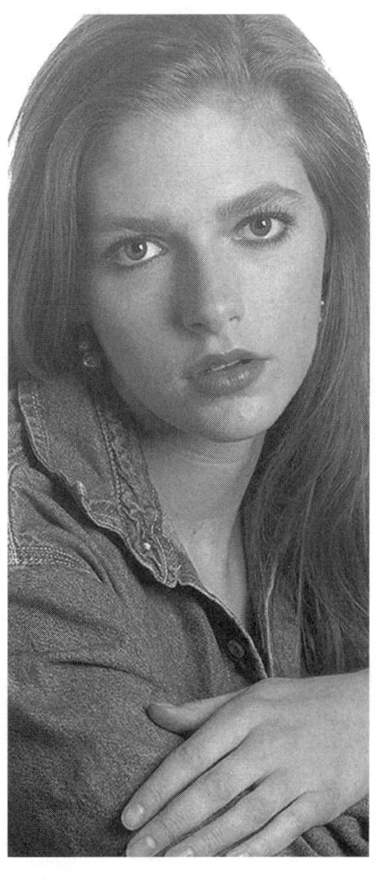

Andy: "She's slept with every guy on the football team."

Parent thinks to himself or herself: *I feel the urge to defend Jessica, but I'll stifle it for now.*

Parent: "Not dating someone who acts like a slut seems important to you."

Notice that you have taken the conversation back to Andy and away from Jessica. He now has the opportunity to identify why he does not want to date someone with loose morals. He has an opportunity to explore the idea that people are not objects, but God's creations.

Andy: "Well, it's important because I respect myself. I wish Jessica had a little self-respect!"

The parent's heart may soar at hearing such a worthwhile value articulated by his or her child. But the parent calmly says: "Andy, I'm glad to hear you talking about self-respect. Where did you get that value?"

Now you get to affirm Andy's spoken value, and you get to name it as a value. That helps your teen in two ways: (1) He receives affirmation as a person and as a Christian. (2) He looks good in front of someone he respects, and the parent gets to respect him. Sounds like a win-win situation all the way around.

Andy: "I don't know. I guess from Sunday school or from you."

Obviously, Christian values have made an impression on Andy. You the parent, the church, and God have all spoken to him.

Tips for Listening

- Teens often speak in code; the code contains their values.

- To open up the code, respond with questions like these:

  "What do you think/feel?"
  "What's your opinion?"
  "What would you do?"

(You may need to ask these questions in several different ways. Just remember who the most important person in the room is. Stay with your teen throughout the dialogue.)

- Give teens a chance to think. Don't rush in with answers.

- Leave fact-finding to another time.

- Stay with your teen. Do not defend the honor or integrity of another person just yet.

- State the Christian value you hear and reaffirm it.

Ten Great Questions to Get Teens to Share More

What do you think about this?
How do you feel about it?
What would you do in this situation?
If you do ________, what could happen? (Ask about possible consequences of specific actions.)
Why do you say that?
What can you do?
How can you help him or her?
You seem upset. (Guess at a particular feeling or emotion. Your teen will correct you if you are wrong.)
What do your friends say?
What are your/their options?

Listening Without Giving In

Too often parents think effective communication means giving in. Giving in usually means that there is no yelling or screaming or slamming of doors. Giving in is an easy, short-term solution. In the long run, giving in does not build faith or values. In the long run, giving in may cause the teen to lose respect for the parent.

Possible Conversations

(1) Teen: "He might be a little old for me."
Parent: "How do you feel about dating someone older than you?"

Does the above exchange constitute permission-giving? No. You are simply giving the teen a chance to explore her own value system. Maybe she will decide for herself that dating an older person is somewhat risky. (Then again, maybe not.)

(2) Teen: "He's so cool, though! Everybody else will be so jealous if I go out with him."
Parent: "*Everybody* wants to date him?"

Your teen may have some doubts about an eighteen-year-old who wants to date a much younger teen. She may question his need to go out with her or her need to go out with him.

If she is not mature enough to have doubts that let you have an opening, then you have to think through your boundaries and attempt to negotiate. Are there any circumstances or boundaries or settings that would be acceptable to you?

(3) Teen: "Can I go out with him?"
Parent: "Why don't you invite him to drop by the house one afternoon so we can meet him first?" OR
"Why not invite him to one of your youth group functions at church?"

Positive communication and careful listening can foster increased reflection and healthy decisions. Let's listen!

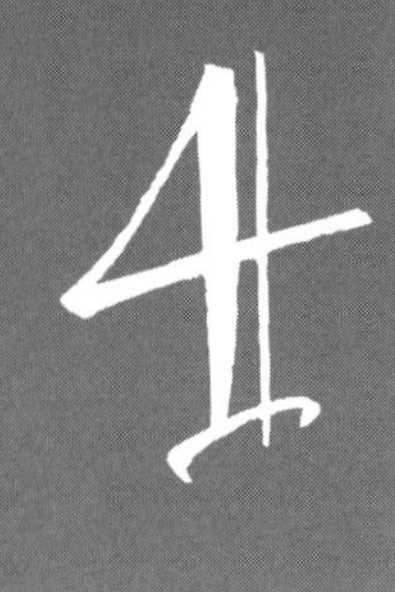

They're in Too Deep! Positive Christian Relationships

God's Say

In the Gospel of John, Jesus passes through the territory of Samaria and engages in conversation with a woman by the well. While the story is about Jesus, the living water, we also discover something about this woman.

"Jesus told her, 'Go and bring your husband.' The woman answered, 'I don't have a husband.' 'That's right,' Jesus replied, 'you're telling the truth. You don't have a husband. You have already been married five times, and the man you are now living with isn't your husband'" (John 4:16-18).

Only Jesus could have known all that about a person after a five-minute conversation. If you or I had been talking with the woman, we might have said, "Woman, could you at least slow down a little bit? Five marriages and now you are in another relationship?" We may fear that our youth will also make poor choices when it comes to relationships, just as the woman by the well did.

Jesus Makes All the Difference

Your teen's relationship with Jesus is crucial when it comes to interacting with others. Jesus knew that relationships are healthiest when they flow from a solid relationship with him. He encouraged the woman at the well to discover such a relationship. In that context she was able to realize that she was important.

Having a relationship with Jesus can ensure that a teen will discover her or his worth as a valued child of God's. In dealings with the opposite sex, youth who have this sense of self-worth will not tolerate being treated as things or objects. They will know instead that they are children of God.

Tips for Listening

Your teen's relationship with Jesus and with you can make a difference

- ▶ when you model a good relationship with your spouse;
- ▶ when your relationship with your teen offers him or her a safe place to explore feelings, faith, and values;
- ▶ when your teen realizes that she or he is a child of God's.

Capture the Moment

Think about how you model good relationships:

1. Do you value and support your partner's work?
2. Do you value your partner's body, or do you view it as an object?
3. Do you value your partner's spiritual life by participating in it or asking about it?
4. Do you participate in your partner's recreational activities?

Now, think about the portrayals of both good and bad relationships that we find in the media.

1. How are people portrayed on TV?
2. What images or advertisements do you see on the freeway as you commute to work?
3. What images do you hear in the music or radio stations that you listen to?

Age Differences in Teens

Sometimes during the promotion of human sexuality events in a local church a parent will say, "My senior high teens went through this course when they were in middle school. They claim they don't need it now."

Wrong! The issues surrounding one's sexuality are more complex in the later teen years than they were in middle school. Older adolescents confront decisions that can lead to the creation of new life or that can result in disease and even death. Relationships at this later age are no longer just about calling persons of the opposite sex on the phone. Relationships now have the potential for including the whole spectrum of of pain and joy.

Generally, the best advice for the parents of younger teens is to stay in the background of the teens' relationships. Let them experience both the fun and the disappointment that relationships can include, unless they cross over into abuse, harassment, or exclusiveness. Hurt feelings as a result of rejection do not constitute abuse. Being rejected is simply part of living in a hurtful world. These beginning relationships can provide a safe place to learn hard and painful lessons.

Your teens will be better served if you rejoice when they rejoice and weep when they weep. Trying to fix a relationship is not your job. Listening to feelings, reflecting those feelings, and reinforcing beliefs and values are your best tools. Taking teens to church and getting them involved in Christian education and a youth group will give them safe places to learn relational skills with responsible and respected adults. Their faith will also be reinforced. Your teen's world will be expanded as he or she turns to other adults for advice and counsel.

Thirteen-year-old teen: "Brittany wants to go out with me! What do I say to her?"

How should a parent respond? Is your youth asking permission or making an announcement? Probably it is an announcement.

Parent: "What does going together mean?"
Teen: "It means we like each other and talk on the phone."
Parent: "How long do most people go together?"
Teen: "Oh, about two weeks."

You sigh with relief. At thirteen "going together"is not a dating situation. Rather, it is a public announcement that the two teens are a couple, for now, in the eyes of others. The relationship may last a week or two months. Letting teens experience the trials and tribulations of "going together" is part of their socialization, of learning to relate to the opposite sex.

The Phone Rings All the Time

A communications explosion confronts today's parents. Is that ringing sound the pager, the cell phone, or the home phone? Often these days it is a female voice asking to speak to your son. Parents are frustrated by the amount of time teens spend on the phone and the number of youth who call their home every day, especially late at night. These calls are the first stages of the socialization of a teen. Phone conversations are how youth learn to talk to the opposite sex. Talking over the phone can be less awkward or threatening than face-to-face conversations in the beginning.

Boundaries still need to be applied. Communicating by phone is important to a teen, but others in the family have rights too. Extending courtesy to other family members and understanding limits is necessary. Boundaries might include a designated time limit on the phone each night, completion of homework before use of the phone, giving up the phone when a parent needs the phone, no calls after 10:00 P.M., or certain times for each child in the family to use the phone.

Modeling a Healthy Relationship

Treating youth as important people of worth, and respecting their feelings, teaches them about relationships. You are modeling healthy relationships.

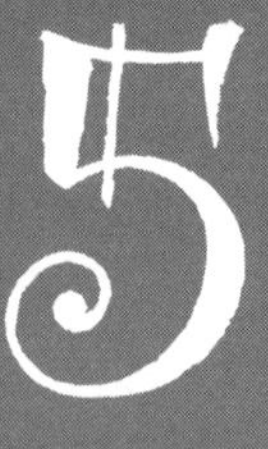

Wait, Wait, Wait It Out!

God's Say

In the Book of Genesis, Joseph has been sold into slavery in Egypt and lives in the home of Potiphar, his Egyptian owner:

"Joseph was well-built and handsome, and Potiphar's wife soon noticed him. She asked him to make love to her, but he refused. . . . 'I won't sin against God by doing such a terrible thing as this' " (Genesis 39:6b-9).

Joseph refused to take advantage of the situation, because he and Potiphar's wife were persons and not just objects for sexual pleasure. Joseph exercised responsibility, self-control, and the ability to avoid the temptation to live just for the moment.

Teens must reject the idea of living just for the moment before they can fully commit themselves to the principle of abstinence. Postponing sexual intercourse until marriage is not just about exercising self-control but also involves an awareness of one's future. The decision to be abstinent can simplify one's life in a number of ways. Those who abstain can avoid worrying about the possible physical consequences of premarital sex as well as possible damage to one's spiritual and emotional health. Abstinence has many more benefits than the fleeting, temporary gratification one might seek in premarital sexual relationships.

Deciding to be abstinent could indeed save your teen's life, in more ways than one. Youth will feel good about themselves and their character when they exercise the values of responsibility, self-control, and not living in the moment for instant gratification.

Reality and Responsibility

Too often, hormones outrace values. Knowing this, a parent may say, "It's better to be safe than sorry." But does this statement give permission for premarital sex? Let's look at that dilemma. How does a parent talk about contraception without giving permission?

The common ground of communication is honest information. Your teen wants to hear the truth from you. Also, when you share the truth with your teen, you are indirectly helping other youth because your teen will become a teacher of others. Honest and accurate information gives your teen a tool for making right and safer decisions about his or her sexuality.

Your teen wants to hear the truth from you.

The speedometer on your car may go up to 120 miles per hour, but you are not likely to drive that fast even once. You resist the temptation to take advantage of the capacity for speed that is available to you. Various kinds of stimuli surround you in your daily environment, but you do not act on all of them because you have a sense of responsibility about the possible consequences of your actions.

Youth also have a sense of responsibility and can make good decisions when given sound, honest information. Parents as well as youth need reliable information to make good, safe decisions. When you as a parent buy or receive a new appliance, don't you expect to get an instruction manual that is clear and accurate? In fact, you would be quite irritated if a manufacturer refused to provide a manual and instead said, "Figure it out for yourself." Such an attitude would be irresponsible on their part.

Your teen's sexuality is a gift. Consider yourself the company that issues the manual on how to regard one's sexuality. Are you going to refuse to provide the manual?

Capture the Moment

Consider these sample conversations with your teen:

Example No. 1: Parent: "I don't want you to have premarital sexual intercourse; but if you make that decision against my wishes, then I want you to use precautions."

Teen thinks to himself or herself: *Wow, my parent just gave me permission to have sexual intercourse*!

OR

"Geez, it's right back on my shoulders."

What would your teen hear in the above example?

Example No. 2: Parent: "Why don't most teens use contraceptives?"

Teen (*possible answers*):

- "They think it will ruin their pleasure."
- "Having contraceptives means you are planning to have sex; that's worse than if it just happens."
- "They don't want to take the time. It might affect the mood."
- "It wouldn't be as romantic."

How would your teen respond to the above question?

Remember when we talked about decision-making and encouraging youth to think for themselves? A conversation about contraceptives underscores the seriousness of even considering engaging in sexual intercourse. A conversation about contraceptives means not leaving everything to one's hormones and the heat of the moment. Your teen will always be faced with temptation. Are you going to give him or her the tools for safe decision-making? Are you going to communicate the values of abstinence and sound, honest decision-making?

When confronted with temptation, Joseph made a decision based on his relationship with God: "I won't sin against God" (Genesis 39:9). Help your teens establish their relationship with God as the firm foundation for making all their decisions. Emphasize the primary values of abstinence and sound, informed decision-making.

Big-Button Issues: How Could I Possibly Talk to My Teen About That!

You have big buttons that your teen can push and set off. How do you talk about sensitive issues with youth? How do you desensitize those buttons? How do you make them smaller?

God's Say

Jesus points out some serious shortcomings on the part of the Pharisees and teachers: "You give God a tenth of the spices from your garden. . . . Yet you neglect the more important matters of the Law, such as justice, mercy, and faithfulness. These are the important things you should have done, though you should not have left the others undone either" (Matthew 23:23).

As parents we get hung up on rules. Our children and youth hear a lot of "don'ts" and "nos" from us: "As long as you are in my house, you will do as I say." Jesus says that our concern should be with "justice, mercy, and faithfulness" rather than with rules. How do justice, mercy, and faithfulness apply to a teen's life, to the youth culture, and to the world as the youth views it?

Our task as parents is to instill moral fiber based on the above qualities. We encourage our teens to take up for a friend who is being gossiped about. We encourage them to stand up for what they think is the right thing to do when others are cheating at school. We encourage them to stand firm when everyone around them is having sexual intercourse, drinking, and doing drugs.

Teens constantly ask, "Why?" They are not content to just accept our views. We will not be around to answer every ethical question or help them confront every situation as they go through life. Other issues will come up that we or society haven't even thought of. Our gift to them is to help them learn how to make good and wise decisions. We give youth chances to practice these skills by not making all their decisions for them. We accept that they will make some poor ones. We help them review their past decisions and pray that they learn from their mistakes. But we continue providing opportunities to enhance their decision-making skills.

Gut Reactions

We react emotionally to sexual issues. It is difficult for us to respond solely from our intellect. We have gut reactions when we hear certain words and phrases. Even stronger feelings surface when we think of these topics in relation to our youth. In these instances, what we know about communicating with our teen can easily go out the window. Our feelings overwhelm our reason, and all the good things we know and have been taught about talking with our teen get shoved to the back of our minds.

When teens bring up big-button issues, they are asking for a non-judgmental arena in which they can discuss the subjects. They care what you think; but even more important, they appreciate your providing a safe environment for discussing these issues. They want to be able to put their thoughts on the table so that they can think through their arguments.

Your Opinion Versus Your Teen's Opinion

Your opinions are not the main concern initially. Those of your teen are. What is behind certain statements on his or her part? What prompted the broaching of a specific topic? If a teen brings up a subject, it means he or she wants a safe arena for discussion. Immediately giving your opinion is not the way to meet that need. Stating your own viewpoint could even end the discussion. Instead, allow your teen to verbalize his or her own views.

Our goal as parents in dealing with big-button issues is honest communication. We desire in-depth conversations with our teens, not just the exchange of a few words or sentences. Teens do want to know your opinion (briefly expressed). But your *first* response does not need to be your own opinion. To keep a discussion going, ask questions. Near the end of the discussion, state your opinion and then ask, "What do *you* think?" Remember that it is OK for the teen to have the last word.

You may believe that certain issues involve not simply opinions but deeply-held values. As a parent you have a right and an obligation to share and defend your values and convictions. Stand firm in your faith. But grant your teen the same privilege you have to form values. As parents we hope that our teens will share our values. We desire to teach those values, but there is a difference between clearly defining one's values and demanding their acceptance by your teen.

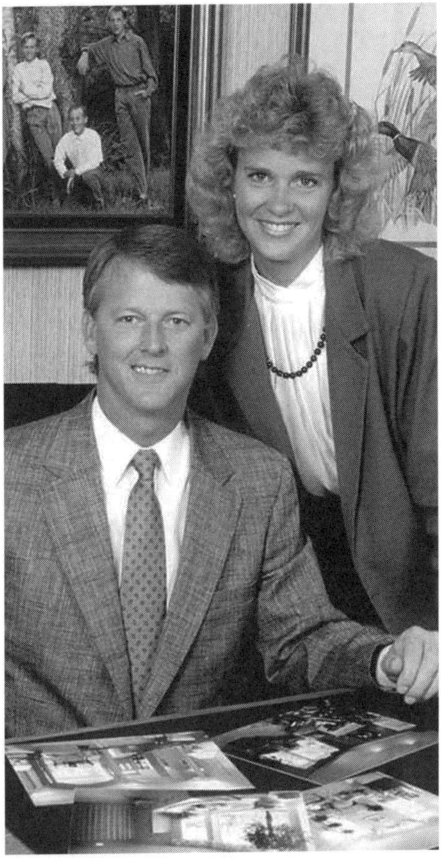

Finally, in some cases you may not have a clearly defined opinion or you may still have doubts about your position. Honesty on your part will help your teens understand that their doubts are OK, too.

Tips for Listening

Remember, when you give your opinion first,

- they might say nothing.
- they might say nothing that contradicts your opinion.
- they might make only statements that back up what you said.
- they might disagree with you and might react angrily.

When you wait, remember

- to ask questions;
- that teens have opinions and values. These ideas belong to them as much as yours belong to you.
- that teens think out loud;
- that what they say now is not their last word. They are growing in their understanding.
- that you may learn something about your teens;
- that doubts are OK;
- that opinions, like a slice of cheese, have two sides;
- that values are deeply held and personal. You and your teens have a right to different values.

TERMS THAT MAY EMERGE IN YOUR CONVERSATIONS:

Abortion

Abortion is removal of the zygote, or fetus, or baby, usually in the first trimester of pregnancy. The words the parent uses to talk about this issue frame the discussion. *Zygote* depersonalizes the act, while *baby* makes it more personal. Which words you choose to use say something about your position on abortion.

Homosexuality

Homosexuality is the preference for sexual or emotional relationships with persons of the same gender. There is no agreement among the scientific, social, psychiatric, and religious communities as to whether homosexual orientation is a genetic trait or an acquired trait. This hotly-debated issue brings forth a great deal of emotion and controversy in many churches.

Some denominations make a distinction between homosexual behavior and homosexual orientation. In the eyes of some churches, homosexual behavior is immoral, while homosexual orientation is not a sin.

Our goal as parents with big-button issues is communication.

Bisexuality

Bisexuality is the preference for relationships with persons of both sexes. Some churches say that bisexuality is incompatible with Christian teaching because it involves homosexual behavior.

Incest

Incest is the term for intimate sexual activity between close relatives. Sexual intercourse is what we usually think of when we use this term. However, other behaviors, such as fondling the genitals or breasts of the other person, might be included. When such activities involve an adult and a child who are related, we may use other terms such as child sexual abuse or molestation.

Incest generally involves the inappropriate use of power and causes confusion about appropriate family roles. One relative usually exerts power over the other person, either emotionally, physically, or financially. Children and teens are persons and not objects. Sexual activity between unequal partners means that the younger person is treated as an object.

Rape

Rape is forced sexual activity (usually intercourse) by someone known or unknown to the victim and against her or his will. Sexual assault that does not include penetration is still unwanted sexual activity. Any person has a right to say "No!" at any point before and during sexual activity. The other person should immediately obey a request to stop; not doing so constitutes rape.

Dating Violence

Dating violence involves emotional abuse, physical abuse, or sexual abuse in a dating or acquaintance relationship. This kind of abuse is a serious crime that is misunderstood and under-reported. Victims of rape, especially rape committed by an acquaintance, often feel responsible and don't report the crime to police. Acquaintance rape is fostered by the common sex-role stereotype that sees men as the aggressor, while women are supposed to be passive and yielding.

Sexual Harassment

Sexual harassment can occur in various workplace and social settings, including schools. This kind of harassment consists of unwanted sexual comments or suggestions or an atmosphere that is sexually offensive to someone. Both males and females may be the victims of sexual harassment. If the offensive activity does not cease after giving fair warning, it should be reported.

Masturbation

Masturbation involves self-stimulation of the genitals, usually leading to orgasm. For the male, stroking the glans and shaft of the penis can produce orgasm. A female may masturbate by rubbing her clitoris or inserting her fingers into her vagina. She may or may not experience orgasm.

Teens pass through puberty ten to fifteen years before marriage is a realistic option, in many cases. Upholding the value of abstinence can mean postponing the experience of sexual intercourse for a number of years. Masturbation can be considered an alternative to sexual intercourse.

Conclusion: Final Exam

- Who's the most important person in the room during a conversation with your teen? (*your teen*)
- What's the most important relationship in your teen's life? (*his or her relationship with God*)
- Who's the most important role model—you, or the media? (*you*)
- What are your most important faith tools? (*the church and the Bible)*
- Will your teen appreciate your efforts to listen and thank you for trying to understand him or her (*yes*)
- Who will be with you in your struggle to be a better parent? (*God*)
- Who will give you the right words to say? (*God*)
- Who loves you? (*God*)
- Who considers you a person of sacred worth? (*God*)
- Who will be with you in your struggle to communicate? (*God*)
- Who forgives you when you fail to do as well as you wish? (*God*)
- Who's the most important person in the room? (*your teen*!)